yoga poems

Books by Leza Lowitz

POETRY
Old Ways to Fold New Paper (1996)

ANTHOLOGIES
A Long Rainy Season (1994)
with Miyuki Aoyama and Akemi Tomioka

Other Side River (1995)
with Miyuki Aoyama

yoga poems

LINES TO UNFOLD BY

LEZA LOWITZ

WITH ILLUSTRATIONS BY ANJA BORGSTROM

Stone Bridge Press • *Berkeley, California*

Grateful acknowledgment is made to the California Arts Council for its generous support in the writing of these poems and to the Spirit Dog Foundation, without whom publication of this book would not have been possible.

The author would like to thank the editors of *Rooms* and *Awaiting a Lover* (Viking-Penguin), in which several of these poems first appeared, sometimes in slightly different form.

The quatrain by Rumi from *Unseen Rain*, translated by John Moyne and Coleman Barks, appears by permission of The Threshold Society (Aptos, California, 1986).

The four-line poems from *Responses Magnetic* (Santa Fe: Katydid Books, 1996) appear by permission of Kijima Hajime.

The figure on the front cover is by Anja Borgstrom and shows the pose *Padmasana* (Lotus). The recurring *om* motif is a stylization of the Sanskrit character and was discovered on a fragment of used wrapping paper.

Published by Stone Bridge Press
P. O. Box 8208, Berkeley, CA 94707
sbp@stonebridge.com • www.stonebridge.com

Text © 2000 Leza Lowitz.
Yoga pose illustrations © 2000 Anja Borgstrom.
Author photo on back cover © 2000 Elaine Fink.

Interior design by Peter Goodman.
Cover design by Linda Shimoda.

Printed in the United States of America.

LIBRARY OF CONGRESS CATALOGING-IN-PUBLICATION DATA
Lowitz, Leza.
    Yoga poems: lines to unfold by / Leza Lowitz; with illustrations
    by Anja Borgstrom.
        p. cm.
    Includes bibliographical references.
    ISBN 1-880656-45-0
        1. Yoga—Poetry. I. Title.

    PS3562.O8963 Y64 2000
    811'.54—dc21

                                              00-025569

contents

The center clears. Knowing comes:
The body is not singular like a corpse,
But singular like a salt grain
still in the side of the mountain.

RUMI

ıntroduction

"Within my body, there's a city." This line came to me one winter evening in 1995 as my head dangled in downward-facing dog and I tried to breathe, remain relaxed, ignore the pull in my hamstrings and pain in my arms. I repeated the line to myself and felt calmer. Two breaths—three, four. I pressed my heels to the ground, felt the earth "a little lighter between my toes." Having just returned from an eight-month trip to Tokyo that lasted five years, the thought of my body containing a city appealed to me. Another foreign city to explore, I thought. An untraveled city. I was ready to go there. My bags were packed.

Although I didn't know it then, I had come back to America greatly changed by my five years in Japan. I was suddenly single, between jobs and worlds. In mellow Northern California, I was still reeling from the pace of Tokyo, where I'd been too busy to deal with my body, my breath, my feelings. I'd rush from one job to another, then another, rush to the gym, then rush out to dinner or a party, rush to catch the last train home, fall into bed, and do it all again the next day. Back in California, stripped of my busy-ness, I was an expatriate in my own skin. Yoga made me take up residence there again.

The journey inward was a personal one, and not always easy. I discovered places in my body that were so root-bound or rock-hard I had to pick at them gingerly because I was very afraid of breaking. In the beginning, I was terrified of breaking my back, breaking my neck. I had no idea how strong I really was, or how weak. When first doing the Plough, I couldn't breathe. In the Fish, I felt as if I was choking. I was very lucky in that my teacher, Veera Wibaux, a mime and a mystic, taught our Hatha yoga class with a sense of play and joy. I learned how to do a headstand, but first, I learned the art of falling. I watched my fears melt, or sometimes not. In the process, I released acres of emotional residue that years of therapy and various forms of healing had chipped away at but not yet unearthed. I'd done aerobics for years, studied martial arts, Tai-Chi, Zen meditation, yet yoga was the one practice that allowed me a deep, meditative experience of my body. Breath by breath, I allowed myself to unfold.

As I deepened my yoga practice, I got out of my own way and let my body move my spirit. As my body and heart opened, so did the channels of creativity. "Downward Dog" was the first poem I wrote, and continues to be one of my favorites. Over the next few years, the poems kept coming. They came in class or at home while I was in the pose, or just after. Other times only a line was born, or a poem would come about a pose I couldn't do. This too, was a lesson. Was it okay to write a poem about a pose I hadn't yet mastered? Wasn't exploration of the pose as important—if not more so—than the execution of a picture-perfect posture? Wasn't it wonderful to embrace failure, to pick oneself up and try again? Most of the time I thought so.

Surprisingly, the magic of going inward also took me away from myself. Breath was the bridge to greater self-understanding, which led to a deeper concern for others and to greater involvement in the community. When I gave public readings, I would demonstrate the posture before I read the poem. Doing so brought the poems more fully into my heart than ever before. The poems came alive for me when

I entered the poses. Conversely, the pose was brought to life by the words, and the sometimes too-serious atmosphere of the poetry reading was lightened. In 1998, I participated in a benefit reading for a local literary newsletter in a small town in West Marin, and an editor-at large for *Yoga Journal* was in the audience. She liked the poem, and her encouragement led me to continue writing these "yoga poems." So this book was born.

The book's structure is an homage to the eight limbs the ancient sage Patanjali described in the *Yoga Sutra*—a revolutionary system of mind and body awareness that the Tibetan master Djwhal Kuhl said ". . . will be used to train disciples in mind control for the next 7,000 years." The eight-limbed yogic practice parallels the eightfold path of early Buddhism, and both practices are considered essential to spiritual development. The eight limbs of Patanjali's *Yoga Sutra* are basically eight cumulative stages toward the "acquisition of yogic power" and include moral principles, observances, posture, breath control, withdrawal of the senses, concentration, meditation, and pure contemplation.

During my practice, I was inspired by the wisdom and depth of the *Yoga Sutra,* and I liked the idea of "sutra" as it relates both to blessing/prayer and to "suture" or stitching. The poems in this book stitch together mind/body /spirit experiences. After all, the word yoga is derived from the Sanskrit *yuj*, to yoke, or join. It is yoking, a coming together of mind and body.

12

Each poem is named after an *asana*, or posture (in Sanskrit and English), or a breathing practice. The poems are arranged under a particular "limb" according to the nature of the experience they describe. Some are directly related to particular asanas, either in concrete or abstract ways, while others are more narrative and personal. Many are abstract "meditations" that surfaced through a highly physical and spiritual yoga practice. Some poses, such as Lunge or Dolphin, are modern variations derived from ancient postures and have no uniformly accepted Sanskrit names. There are many more postures and breath exercises than the poems in this book cover. And, since breath is the heart of yoga and is central to every posture, some poems in the Pranayama ("Breath Control") section are named for postures rather than breathing exercises.

Many yoga poses are named after animals, and as such, are inherently provocative. Eagle, Peacock Tailfeather, Frog, Cobra. The shape and energy of the poses themselves are rife with metaphorical associations. In the Bridge pose, we build a bridge with our backs to carry ourselves through transitions, rising to life's challenges with strength and support. We find our center of balance in the Tree pose, embracing our inner poise despite the winds of change that threaten to bend or break us. We welcome the turn of the day in our Sun Salutations, honoring the sun's healing rays and making them one with our own, embracing the outer light and bringing it in, radiating. Inverted poses such as Headstand flip us upside down, literally turning things on their heads. Yet, we must find equilibrium and embrace our fear of the unknown. What would life be like if we never took risks—never tried headstand or handstand in the first place? What might we miss by backing away from the exploration of something we did so freely as children?

As I moved in and out of the eight "limbs" or stages of yoga practice, which are not successive or absolute, the poems became less about struggle and personal history or reflection, and more about acceptance, opening, unity, and connection. The eight limbs themselves reflect a movement from separateness to unity, and so did my practice. I found that yoga gave me patience, took me away from the focus on the "goal" and into a deeper appreciation of the "process," away from "doing" and into "being." Yoga moved me away from thinking and into pure experience, into trust and sometimes complete joy. The record keepers of the universe know the value of listening. I listened to my body, then I let it be. Some of the more narrative poems are a record of what came up in the stillness—what I embraced, and what I let go of. These poems are grouped in their own section entitled "The Unfolding," because they constitute a personal journey toward acceptance and forgiveness.

Embracing the "process" rather than the "goal" was extremely beneficial to me in the creative process as well as in life. Over the past few years, I have been writing a novel. Learning to accept where I was, to enjoy where I was at that moment (even if I was "stuck") and not think about where I wanted to be next year, was a very valuable lesson to me. I wanted to put some blank pages in this book so that when you invite your own yoga poems to emerge, they have a comfortable place to land.

Yoga Poems can go anywhere yoga goes. Teachers can read the poems aloud in class during meditation periods, while students are in the actual pose, or during restorative classes. Or they can be read privately, alone. The book is as individual as your yoga practice—or mine. Although there are many disciplines of yoga, I enjoy Hatha yoga. My practice alternates between Iyengar and Kripalu styles, which for me invite a slower, deeper, exploration of the psyche and spirit, augmented by a weekly practice of the challenge and vigor of Ashtanga yoga.

* * *

A few years into my new life, I married a Japanese man I considered my soul-mate, who moved from Tokyo to California and changed his life, too. We bought a funky 1930s bungalow in a small coastal town thirty minutes from anything. We adopted an abandoned dog and taught her how to play in the waves. I put a sign up in the post office for anyone interested in yoga classes. I had two calls—one from a woman who had five friends interested in yoga classes, the other from a woman who had six. Soon I had up to seventeen students. Where was the teacher? I had to grow into the role. Six years later, I am still a beginner. But, after all, gifts don't wait to be given. They come when they're ready. So this book came to me. And now I give it to you, with love and light.

acknowledgments

Hands clasped in gratitude to my first yoga teacher, Veera Wibaux, whose humor, grace, and spiritual guidance opened up a whole new world, and to:

Jill Minye of The Open Hand in Sebastopol for inspiring me to go deeper and inviting me to be wider, John Smith for compassionate teaching and beautiful poetry read during practice, Ganga White and Tracey Rich for helping me bring the healing warmth of the sun and the subtle mysteries of the moon to my practice and teaching, B. K. S. Iyengar for passing on the tradition, and the venerable Krishnamacharya for coming first and lighting the way.

A thousand rays of light to Abigail Davidson, Les Berkowitz, and the Santa Fe Boss Dogs for big licks of inspiration and an ever-deepening, ever-magical friendship, Richard Ruben for the same (plus twenty years of the best phone calls anyone could dream of), and Nina Zolotow for her friendship and decade-long unerring sense of the brave and the true. This book could not have happened without each of you.

I owe CB Follett and Ralph McCarthy much for their support of my writing and insightful reading of the manuscript, Anja Borgstrom for her wonderful images, Don Best for seeing the potential and being unafraid to manifest it, Cullen Curtiss, Olivia Weber, Yurika Kimijima, Shizuko Angel, Rick DeNoble, and especially Peter Goodman for sharing the enthusiasm and supporting the vision.

I'm fortunate to have Rob Brezsny and Sue Miller pointing the way, and I'm so grateful to the Dillon Beach/Petaluma Yoga Circle—Alexis, Azar, Carolyn, Connie, Ellen, Eva, Helene, Ingrid, Jan, June, Laurinda, Mary Ann, Megg, Melanie, Milton, Roberta, Ruth, Sandra, Sharon, Sue, Ted, Theresa—for being the best students I could ever wish to learn from. I'd also like to thank Beverly Sikes for giving such beautiful form to my poems.

Alison Anderson, Miyuki Aoyama, Jeff Berner, Chris Blasdel, David and Elin Chadwick, Elaine and Mark Fink, Jack and Adelle Foley, Lynn Freed, Molly Giles, Kyle Glenn, Edgar Honetschlager, Ed and Chako Ifshin, Daissy and Ralph Koch, Robert Kushner, Helene Leff, Michelle Lizieri, John Mason, Janet and Jim Moore, Christoph and Nicola Niedermair, Elizabeth Ogata, Fumi Oketani, Lily Pond, Angelo Proserpi, Lucas Reiner, Donald Richie, Nancy Roberts, Elliot Schain, Stuart Siegel, Harold Silen, Amy Skezas, Mihoko Sugiura, Joan and Helen Taschian, Andrea Taylor, Amy Trachtenberg, Bo Wiley, Maud Winchester, and my family sustained me with their belief in my ability to bend but not break.

I'm blessed that Tom Centollela and Anne Cushman lead my "Downward-Facing Dog" out of the pack, and that my wild dog Aska shows me daily how it's done.

Finally, *namaste* to Shogo Oketani for providing much-needed balance, love, and open arms to catch me whenever I fell. I dedicate this book to you.

L.L.

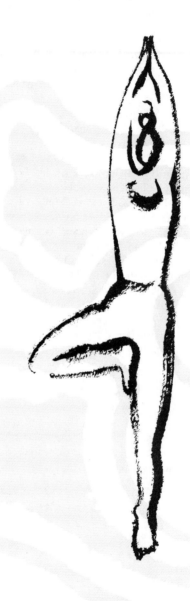

Vrksasana

TREE

yama

MORAL PRINCIPLES

Adho Mukha Svanasana

DOWNWARD-FACING DOG

Within my body
there's a city—

nameless streets
dead-end alleys

of pains and promises,
a mapless Atlantis

cordoned off
by years and bones.

The muscles pull
the tendons throb

my joints crack out
their resistance—

places I've ached
undetected

for a quarter of a century
send out their muted frequencies

from an unfamiliar
pose.

Descending too quickly,
I implode.

Down here, or even up there
breath is the most

difficult of absences
and so, two finger-widths

into the *hara*
I find my bearings

mind-body-belly
oxygen tank both empty and full.

Listen to the place
you feel it the most

says the teacher,
head dangling from

adho mukha
svanasana

a single bulb
on a simple cord.

So once again
I go down deeper

to where
the muscles pull

the tendons throb
the pain travels

21

its clandestine escape
and then retreats

in the halfway reach
where each breath

razes another
skyscraper I've aspired to,

brings the earth up
a little lighter between my toes.

Kurmasana

TORTOISE

Moving hard-backed through life
the enigma of a destination
never a cause for worry.
Mottled shell concealing
the being beneath,
thoughts buried like eggs in the sand
future unhatched
in the slow-moving sea
the tangled seaweed of a schedule
unknown.
Here, arms float on each side
parting the waves of resistance.
An ocean in my veins,
floating world in my watery skin
head looking out for voyage
heart looking in to Goddess
womb of earth that bore me
and cast me out
once and forever
into the soup.

Virabhadrasana II

WARRIOR II

Here there is nothing to fight
except willfulness.
Some lean too far
into the past.
Others stretch way out
into the future.
The true warrior
stays in the
moment,
burning deeper
into whatever comes,
or sometimes with
even more difficulty,
what doesn't.

Padangustha Dhanurasana

BOW

For woman,
bow is both
noun and verb.

How to bend
without breaking?
How to tie a ribbon
around a life
without constriction?
How to stretch
and not snap?

How to love?
How to live?

Happy Baby / Dead Bug

One at the beginning of its life
the other at the end—
one at the top of the food chain
the other, the bottom—
coming together
in the shape
and the name of the pose.

In Bangkok I saw a man
gather flies to feed his child.
The child ate them and smiled.

26

Krauncasana

HERON

Still as silence
what I hold in this life
is thousands of years of DNA,
the mystery of a moment
in which what falls away
is effort
and what changes
is everything
that grows longer
and stronger,
joyous
in flight.

Vrksasana

TREE

How difficult it is
to stand straight and tall.
How much more difficult
to do it on one leg.
God knew what she was doing
when she made us bipedal.
Yet we spend most of life
hunched over,
denying the true weight
of the gift we've been given.
Now the trunk aches
as it tries to expand to full height—
buried, as it's been,
in the bone.
Gain and loss
victory and defeat
fame and shame
body and mind
mind and soul—
dualities vanish.
The tree grows green
against the blue sky,
drawing the sun's rays
through the slatted shutters
of the ribs.
We are the roots.
We are the forests and the trees.
Here, there is only one trunk.
On it rests the world.

Urdhva Mukha Svanasana

UPWARD-FACING DOG

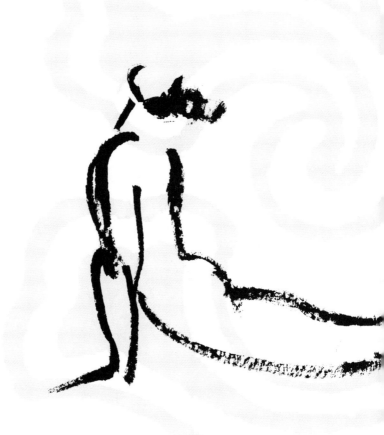

niyama

OBSERVANCES

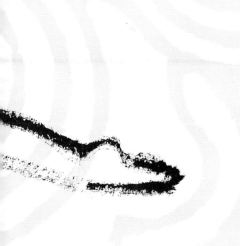

Matsyasana

FISH

Open the heart
and the heart opens you—
salt of the creator
eye of the beholder
stretch your arms overhead
receive
the rainfall of pure clarity
and let it
come down.

Surrender to the boundless
earth, sea, and sky
place them like a garland
around the altar of a life,
seal
a prayer for peace
at its base,
swim
in its mysteries,
unafraid of sinking.

Open the heart
and the heart opens you.

Lunge

Map of the sky
in the mirror of the eye
a universe expands.

How to honor this great leap?
Sing, in the wild blue wilderness
of the river of blood
flowing in your veins.

Open your mind
close your eyes
trust the path you are on.
Terra incognita
always means
that first awkward step
of surrender.

Urdhva Mukha Svanasana

UPWARD-FACING DOG

My dog is an alpha female,
otherwise known as an alpha bitch
my dog is as smart as a fox
as beautiful as a jaguar
and slightly demented.
My dog is a she-wolf
tough and crafty
with a touch of the warrior
in her blood.
My dog is as sweet as clover
loves to have her tummy rubbed,
takes over the couch and
digs up newly planted gardens.
Who says she doesn't
resemble her owner?
My dog is
sometimes very beautiful
sometimes very strange looking
sometimes downright ugly.
My dog is a mutt.
My dog is me.
My dog is you.
My dog is almost human.
My human is almost dog.
She likes beta males to chase her,
alpha males to wrestle down
and alpha females,
but only if they are younger
or about the same age.
She fights other bitches
who look at her the wrong way
and will win 99% of the time,

34

a K-9 trainer said.
My dog was abandoned as a newborn,
lived in a pit for six months
and knows how to survive.
My dog cries whenever I leave
and smiles when I return.
Despite anything I say about her
my dog just *is*,
embodying
everything
I'm trying to live up to:
unconditional love.

Pinca Mayurasana

PEACOCK TAILFEATHER

When you've perfected
this posture
throw it away—
a peacock cannot see
the beautiful feathers
behind it.

Parivritta Janu Sirsasana

REVOLVING KNEE TO HEAD

Deep in the ground
a root grows out of nothing.
Soon, a blossom emerges
sending its fragrance
to the wind.
A bee stops for supper.
Pollen spawns an offshoot,
years later
a garden of verbena appears.
All that lives grows within.
All that dies lives within.
Each breath nurtures
an unfolding,
pours water
to a budding blossom
and the chest flowers open
breath by breath,
leaning toward spring.

Karnapidasana

I was almost married to dispassion.
Then I had a lover
who unearthed
the light of limb and breath,
in the tremor and warmth of flesh
he made my body grow.

Out of stone sprung a paradise
from the cold concrete surface,
108 earthly desires
bloomed deep in the tongue.
Tangled in the numinous places
we would kill the numb weeds
that died happily in each other's fists,
each time finding another way
to assassinate what strangled the soul.

Skin sliding over skin
like snails over wet leaves
the sticky compass of the hips
rotating until the limbs themselves
became unhinged.

We buried flesh in flesh,
closed off the world
and the darkness disappeared.

This is the only life I've ever known.
Take it, he said, *there will be another.*
Gentle Lazarus, you were wrong.
So now with ear to knee,
I rake each pebble

of my body back to me,
for each season something dies
and something new springs
from the soil of a garden
that cultivates the aura of the temple
long after it has crumbled,
seeding something new
for the sacred
for the poem
for the heart
brought back to life
by the lover
whose touch is found
in the unfolding
like an answer buried
deep within the ground.

Sukhasana

CROSS-LEGGED POSE

Like an archeologist
I believe that somewhere
in this dark old cave
I'll find a worthy treasure,
and I do,
lifting my sternum
stretching out sacrum, lumbar, psoas, iliacus
dusting off these mythical
shards of me,
names like an ancient language,
hieroglyphic prayer
I'm learning by heart.
Pulling them out,
I find another path
to a hidden chamber
and another
and another.
When the rock chips
and clears
all these riches
are visible—
and I'm just sitting,
digging deeper,
blowing off the dust.

40

Ardha Chandrasana

HALF-MOON

She lifts her leg in the air.
The standing one shakes
ready to sprint for the door
buckle under the pressure
simply crumble and fall.

She remembers to breathe
lifts her leg just a bit higher
imagining the moon poised on her toes,
shining on dreams in a present unknown.

She holds her leg steady
thinks: *this is my life*
there's no one watching.
This leg is a blade of grass
containing fields.
Let them blow
gently in the wind.

Something within pivots
on a single breath.
Yes, this is my life, she thinks
and finds

this is
just the
right moment
to die.

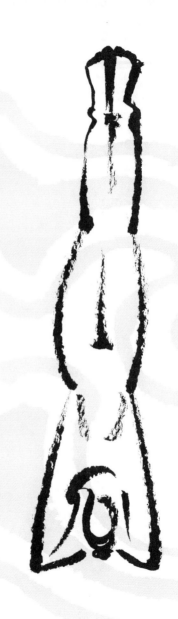

Sirsasana

HEADSTAND

asana

POSTURE

Sirsasana

HEADSTAND

Morning light rises across the dark room
like the sun up over the ocean.
Forming a cup with my palms
I pour my head into it,
let my legs spill against gravity,
uncurling toward the sky.
Standing the world on its head
everything I know is upended.
What I believed was inevitable—
what I once thought was solid
what I perceived as impossible—
the map of certainties
drawn on the sand of life
upturns in the tide.
King of all asanas,
everything is right where it should be
when the crown of my soul
rests blissfully in my palms
and I'm born
head-first to the world again,
like the sun over the Pacific,
taking my time
to rise.

Paschimottanasana 6

If I learn the truth in the evening
I can die in the morning,
Confucius said.
But which evening?
Which morning?
Which truth?

If I die in the morning
will I be reborn
in the evening?
If the truth I learn turns out
to be a lie,
do I get to live anyway?

If the lie I learn
turns out to be the truth
and I am already dead
where does that leave me
tonight and tomorrow?

Nothing to do but surrender.

Whatever thought you just had . . .
the teacher says in the midst of
the pose,
. . . name it.

45

Bakasana

CRANE

It's easy to fall
in a hall of mirrors,
mistake the moon on the water
for the moon itself.
It's easy to get stuck
in the minus-tide banks
of the muddy mind
and stay there forever
afraid of having to fly.
It's easy to loot the heart
for its last honest beat
but the toes know
the difference
an inch of solid ground
can make,
the arms know
that the wavering heart
opens to an endless marsh,
and the fingers know
to spread their tips into wings
when the cage door opens
and the bottom
          falls
out.

46

Adho Mukha Vrkasana

HANDSTAND

one by one
    legs scissor in the air
        for a moment holding
           against gravity
                then in another moment
                falling

one by one
    it's fear that pulls the legs down
        makes it all the more beautiful
           when the parts spin
                together in one wind

one by one
    two legs finally
           united against waiting
        for a better time
           to take the leap.

47

Chakravakasana

A hundred stray cats
and I am the one
who lands on the fence,
arching my back
awakening the fishbone within.
My scratchy tongue
loses its roughness
my high-pitched hiss
softens into song.
Recalling the movement of fish
I spring into action,
each unknown alley
suddenly a river
rushing for me.

Bhujangasana

COBRA

Shedding my skin
    skinning my shreds
        leaving behind
            every failure
                every success
                    every anger
                            ever expressed
                          or never expressed.
                What's left behind
            stays behind,
        its ancient
    poisonous sting
all but forgotten.

Ardha Matsyendrasana

LORD OF THE FISHES

This is one pose I cannot do.
Once Lord Siva went to a lonely island
and explained to Parvati
the mysteries of Yoga.
A fish near the shore
heard everything.
It remained still, concentrating.
Siva sprinkled water on it.
Instantly, the fish took divine form.
The Lord of the Fishes,
now a God,
spread knowledge of Yoga.

This is the pose I cannot do.
Sometimes I cannot even
be a human being.
How then,
can I become God?
I was born from water
and when I die
will return
to water too.

Ujjayi Pranayama

VICTORIOUS BREATH

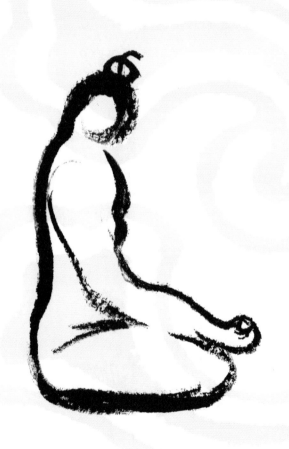

pranayama

BREATH CONTROL

Gomukhasana

COW-FACED POSE

Many times we reach
for what we cannot see.
yet we fail to grasp it.
Many times we have been unaware
that our breath has not ended,
and if we do not know
how many times
our breath has saved us
we need only to listen
to the beat of the heart
today.

A drowning man reaches for a lifesaver.
A lifesaver exists
only for a drowning man.
If your lungs have not filled with water
you are not drowning.
So why are you still reaching?

You do not need a lifesaver.
Just remember to breathe.

Sanmukhi Mudra

SIX-MOUTH BREATHS

Who owns the wind?
Who owns my breath?
These impossible riddles
haunt me.

Turning into the wind
the wind turns into me.
Those possible answers
keep me breathing.

Uttanasana

STANDING FORWARD BEND

Mind, mind
how much you want to say
am I doing it right?
can I stay here long enough
or even a second longer
can I eat an ice cream sandwich
after class,
oh, but will class ever end?
Mind,
will you ever shut up?
will my legs stop shaking?
will my head reach lower?
Will I
can I
should I
could I
let go of my mind
listen to my breath
listen through my breath
let it move through this body
reach out to this moment,
this world,
this life,
      & let it go?

Ujjayi Pranayama

VICTORIOUS BREATH

Slow and deep
into the heart of the day.
With each inhalation
comes an exhalation
twice as long.
Slow and deep
filling the lungs
with infinite space,
the sun rises and sets
in each single breath.
Forget about tomorrow.
Now is an eternity
and life is a victory
so celebrate
the heart of the day.

57

Dolphin

What a big drink of life
I take with my in-breath
before diving into the sea.
What a big drink of life
I let out in a burst,
rising from the waves.
Traveling the world's oceans
I carry the pattern of the tides within.
Underwater rhythms make up my heartbeat
the song of the ocean sings in my skin,
calling the waters home.
And so it is with me.

Riding the waves
surf curling at my edges
I dive into the deep reefs of time.
Drenched by the ocean blue
the sound carries me
in leaps and bounds
out from the depths
and back into the wild,
wet world.

Siddhasana

INSPIRED SEER

We sit
legs bent
eyes half-closed
to the world.

We go down
to the hallway
of beginning,
working deep
from the bone.

Breathing
is living.
Sitting
clears the mind
of all things.

But where do they go?
Into
the circle of earth
beneath us,
into
the center
within.

No place is too small
for the sacred.

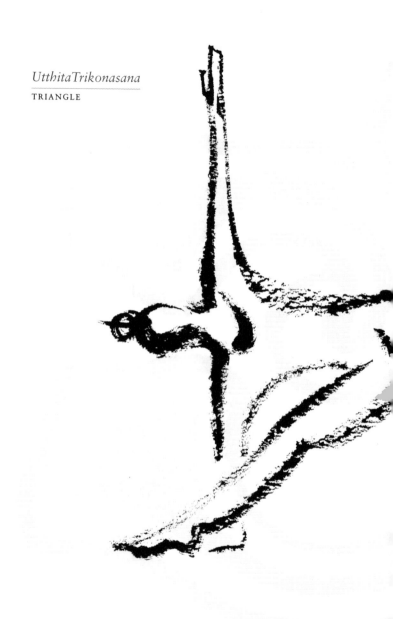

Utthita Trikonasana

TRIANGLE

pratyahara

WITHDRAWAL
OF THE SENSES

Simhasana

Queen of the jungle,
she knows no fear.
In goes the holdingholdingholding
out goes the tongue
fingers, eyes, head, breath
everything reaching
for more space
in which to roam.

Bharadvajasana

SEATED SIDE TWIST

A child balancing on a seesaw
an eagle falling from its nest
before first flight,
always a chance
for a new beginning
on an ordinary afternoon,
another way to
become immortal
within the mortal,
to hear the breath
within the breath.

Throwing anything away
is freedom—
caution to the winds.

Turning to face the god within,
first crying, then laughing
like a child.
In the twist,
life realigns.
Something is released
from the soul,
something more
yearns for release
from the heart,
and even this wall
has wheels.

63

Urdhva Dhanurasana

WHEEL

Rolling on the earth
forever turning,
churning
changing.
A life,
the seasons,
this world.
A word about reinvention:
if only man
could learn
to
stop
where he is.

64

Salabhasana

I dreamt of Quan Yin's eyes,
entering Quan Yin's eyes
always open, every direction.
I fell into the tunnel of her gaze,
became a locust and hopped away.

I dreamt I was floating on a lotus leaf
eating bits from beneath me,
then I was speeding down
the highway
flashing red lights behind me
and when the cop
pulled me over
he retrieved
Miles Davis' dripping trumpet
from my hood,
held it out to me like a chrysanthemum
together we sipped tea made from its leaves.

I dreamt I was hopping
in the wheatgrass of the world
carrying the plague of love.
What a wonderful dream!

I never had such dreams before.
Or if I did, I woke up
too late to remember them.
Now I keep a journal on my bedstand
like an invitation to strange visions,
and they come
in all shapes and sizes
and I let them.

65

Setu Bandasana

BRIDGE

In her dream, there's a bridge,
always a bridge.
In the dream, she runs on the pavement between cars,
ephemeral body, feet never touching the ground.
She has no armature of steel,
no four-wheel drive or emergency brake.
Only a thin black dress, pale white skin,
hair flowing like a wild flame
engulfing the pavement behind her.
Dog, skunk, possum & deer
die in the dark speed of daylight
but this is no place for a woman
of soft flesh and strong bosom.
For many years, she couldn't drive over a bridge.
Then she conquered her fear
by rolling up the windows
and screaming in the glass distance of her throat
until the scream sailed out into a laugh and died.

Leaving her body, she surveyed the steel passage:
looking from above, she believed
she could soar over its ribs.
She met a man and got married.
From below, the hard wings of the bridge
spanned out and she saw it as a trap.
She got divorced.
The difference between bridge and bride
is one letter and a lifetime of crossings.
On the ground, it laughs at her
and now she laughs back,
that two-footed bundle of fear radiating

66

blue hemispheres of doubt
now behind her like distant headlights.

For a time she wanted to jump.
Then she found a lover who told her:
the dream of falling is always followed
by awakening.

After you make the inevitable
hard landing,
you get to be alive
in a great big beautiful bed.

67

UtthitaTrikonasana

TRIANGLE

A candlestick with several hands
Reminds me of Kannon,
The thousand-handed
Goddess of Mercy.

Goddess of Mercy
who so many hands,
when holding out just one
would be enough?

Eka Pada Rajakapotasana

ONE-LEGGED KING PIGEON

William Carlos Williams
wrote poems
on a notebook
small enough to fit
in his breast pocket
on his medical rounds.

Yasunari Kawabata
wrote stories
small enough to fit
in the palm of the hand.

The body writes stories
small enough to fit
in the tiniest cell.
Every centimeter
has a different beginning
and end.
Day by day
the gap between
beginning and end
thigh and floor
heel and head
closes up,
the narrative writ large
on each small movement.

69

Start small and the world expands
as Goethe said, but start anyway.
In beginnings
there is the magic
of *yes*.

Hanumanasana

MONKEY

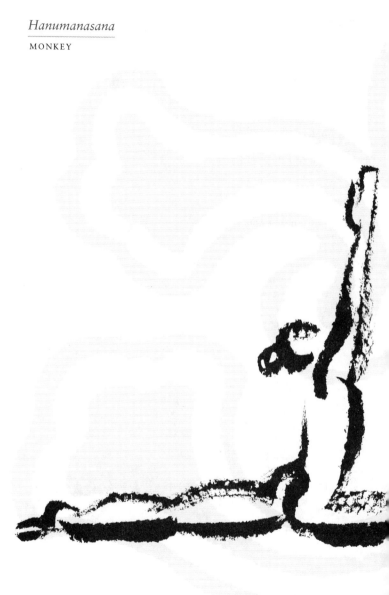

dharana

CONCENTRATION

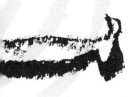

Virasana

HERO

I remember Ryoanji—
how I sat for days at the Kyoto temple,
stared at the sea of pebbles
imagining them into shapes
rocks becoming islands
a mother tiger and her cubs
ships lost at sea
thoughts in the swirling mind
planets swimming around the sun
then finally just rocks
the rectangle of pebbles
walled in by mud, grass, and clay
a reflecting pool for humanity
and nothing but nothing
answering back.
And it didn't matter.
I looked at the lone figure
sitting on the smooth wooden stairs
next to me, and he
looked at me wordlessly
and understood.

In the ancient garden
the questions were a thousand years old
yet the Japanese didn't appreciate Ryoanji
until a German architect studied it,
praised the odd rock garden
hummed the song sung out of tune,
rocks ringing out meaning and no-meaning
in the thousand travelers' faces.

Sitting on my knees
remembering Ryoanji
the thousand faces of the hero
echoing in the distant notes
of a foreign language
returning to me in memory,
and I'm stronger
because of them,
here at home.

Lolasana

In the corner of the room
there's a ball of dust
In the corner of my mind
there's a ball of worry
In the corner of my body
there's a ball of pain
In the corner of the city
there's a ball of traffic
In the corner of the world
there's a ball of confusion
In the corner of the galaxy
there's a ball of light
In the corner of the ball of light
there's a ball of earth
In the ball of earth
there's a world
and a city
and a body
and a mind
and a room
and a ball of dust
multiplied by thousands
swinging back and forth!
Circle of nothingness!
When I think I'm special
it's only because
for a moment
I can see this.

74

Hanumanasana

MONKEY

The story goes like this: The Monkey Chief Hanuman met Rama—the 7th incarnation of Vishnu—when Rama's wife Sita was kidnapped and taken by bandits to Lanka. Hanuman set out for the jungles of Ceylon with an army of monkeys and bears, built a bridge of stones across the sea, and leapt across it to slay Sita's captors and rescue her. But the story doesn't end there. Then he took a deep breath, gathering energy for more heroics to come, since Rama's brother Laksmana had been struck by an arrow and the only cure was the extract of a Himalayan herb. Hanuman sprung back into action, taking one prodigious leap across the sea to the Himalayas. Soon, he returned carrying the elixir that brought Laksmana back to life. Monkey saved both Vishnu's wife and brother by a leap and a bound, and that is only the beginning of the story. So Monkey Chief, please jump from my monkey mind to carry me over the gulf in my split.

Salamba Sarvangasana

A man went to the moon

        not long after I was born.

  Not a woman.

          Why?

  There was the argument of composition

             and then of gravity,

the looming

    possibility

        she wouldn't come down

and of course the fact that lately

        the world itself seems to have lost its form

            contains nothing to jump off from

               is both start and finish

like Escher's hand being born out of paper

          holding a pen

being drawn by another hand

  holding another pen

      and being born from the paper

    the other has drawn.

          One person might be climbing stairs

another is going down on,

    each in the same (or different) directions

and besides, floor and ceiling are meaningless

once the spaceship is in orbit,

and anyway, the sight of land

(moon, volcano, mountain, earth) would raise

the question of ownership,

might move her into asking

whose

name

it

would

bear.

77

Behkasana

FROG

Frog slipped in the mud
and was unable to right himself.
He kicked his legs to the sides
flinging mud into his eyes
first unable to move,
now unable to see.
He knew his lily pond
was just out of reach.
Look what you've done to me!
he croaked to the breeze.

78

Chaturanga Dandasana

FOUR-LIMBED STAFF POSE

Meeting the edge
of the world
kissing the map of possibility
spread out beneath.
Meeting the edge
of the world
breathe in,
as deep
as the earth is deep
breathe out
as steep as the precipice.
Hold your gaze
on the unknown
hold it
know it
because it knows you
and holds you
feel neither fear
nor wonder
just the space between
what was and
what could be.
Greet the edge.
Go over it.
Then feel
for a moment
just what is.

79

Sïrsa Padasana

SCORPION

the tail to the head—
at last, the season has come
all things must connect

Savasana

CORPSE

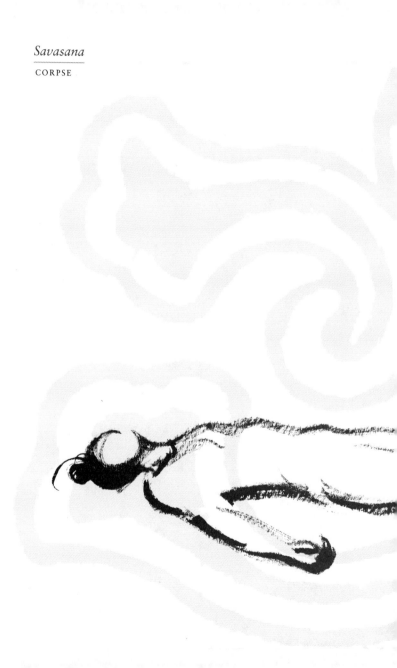

dhyana

MEDITATION

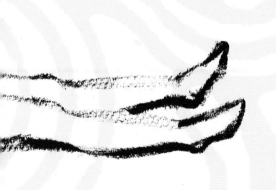

Tadasana

MOUNTAIN

This is the place
the journey begins.
Half rooted in the earth,
half floating in the endless sky.
What would it be like
to be the mountain?
The air is perhaps thinner,
though the sky is not always clear.
The view is sometimes shrouded in fog
sometimes in plain and glorious sight,
but the ascent or descent can kill.
The earth is stable
or sometimes not.
So it is
at base or summit,
yet the mountain never asks
why or for what purpose
it exists.
This is the one difference
between the climber
and the climbed.

Ustrasana

CAMEL

In this desert
resistance crumbles
like sand
through the fingers,
she sleeps
without rest
or water
eyes open
to endless arid days,
face whipped
by each grain of sand
music of the nomad
echoing in the wind
weight of the sky on her back.
In this desert
she sinks to her knees,
wants to be like the camel
sinking deeper still
into the endless sand dune
of time
stretching out
ahead and behind
vast as the desert,
twice as old.

Savasana

CORPSE

Behold, The Dead
teacher of The Dreamer
whose lessons take a
lifetime to learn.
One third of our lives
spent in the night
yet we have trouble
embracing the darkness
in ourselves.
Outside,
sheep sleep under the stars
worms sleep under the earth
mindless of
insomnias &
nightmares.
Inside,
we sleep under
the illusion
of daybreak,
oblivious to
the light.

Supta Virasana

Down on my knees
I peel back the layers of the world.
Nothing left to do
but embrace everything
as it is.
I want to live,
but when I die
I want my funeral to be
like this
and for everyone to bring a sunflower,
bright yellow face
to offer up above.
I want them to shower
my path with light
and send the tall sky
a flower worthy of beholding
and if I gave them anything at all
approaching the gifts they gave me
I want my friends to wash away the sadness
and my enemies to know
I thank them for helping me
never break the promise
of being true to myself.
I want my funeral
to start right now
with a celebration of my life,
proof that everything
in this world—
no matter how broken—
can be transformed.

87

Padmasana

LOTUS

Om mani padme hum
no harm from the invisible world
poets wrote,
sages chanted.
Could it be
the times I was
attacked on the playground
thrown into the bushes
held up at gunpoint
held down to be raped
were indeed visible,
and I might have seen
them coming
if I'd known how
to open my eyes?
But I did not.

I still have a hunger
for the truth.
I'm still looking
for the safe road back home.
The dreams still live within.
Why, after all I've been through,
it's a mystery.
The world still
has its ways
and so do I.
So now I am here,
chanting *om*
casting off
making invisible,
holding but not being beholden to

all that has harmed me
and helped me
grow free.

Threading the Needle

Untangling a knot
that is my life
the knot becomes my teacher.
Gathering the threads into one,
unraveling the closed-up space
a glimmer of light
surfaces between strands.
The needle that is sharp
at dawn
might be broken by dusk.
The thread
that is straight today
doesn't know
it will be knotted tomorrow.
The knot
that is tangled today
could be woven into gold
ten years from now.
That is why
I thread the needle,
honoring the odds
steadying my arms
softening my breath
working the knot,
trusting.

Viparita Karani

SUPPORTED INVERTED POSE

Flipping through the pages
of life's diary
we come to
this day
& the next
& the next.

Open yourself
to the world
and life writes itself
on the heart.

> Close your eyes,
> look inside
> and read its poetry
> again and again
> slowly
> then share it with someone else.

Your neighbor
is you.

Balasana

CHILD'S POSE

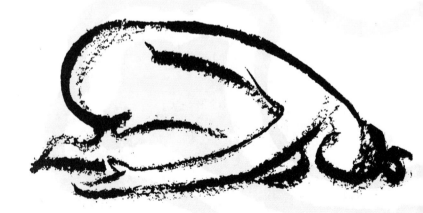

samadhi

PURE
CONTEMPLATION

Ardha Navasana

BOAT

There are two perfect
shapes in the world
a man once said:
the hull of a boat
and a violin.
He might have been a poet
or a painter, and he
might have added a third:
a woman's body.
The hull balances
the boat at sea,
the violin sings
its notes above
the crest of instruments.
A woman's body
moves
where it takes her—
how she sings
when it rides the waves.

Paschimottanasana

SEATED FORWARD BEND

Monk in the snow
lizard on a rock
bee in a flower
stream in a mountain pass
kiss on long-missed lips.

Oh body,
bury me in such perfections
and call them
a soul.

95

Baddha Konasana

BOUND ANGLE

If you could call it perfection
what would it look like?
How would you know it,
feel it,
be it?

Wherever you are now
call it perfection
and know
that in this moment
it is really enough.

Virabhadrasana III

WARRIOR III

Here hangs
a lantern from each side of the body—
one illuminating life
the other death.

In the end
there is only the center
lit up,

only
light
to choose.

Balasana

CHILD'S POSE

Plunging
into the river of joy
diving deeper and wider
within this wraparound life
reborn in the body
as a smile
reborn
in the breath
as radiant light
reborn in the space
between pose and repose
rocking
in infinity—
embracing the union of all that is
and will be.

Garudasana

EAGLE

Before I had a name
I existed in the world
as breath
as the wind
as a star.
For a moment
if I could be the breath
& the wind
& the nameless star
I'd meet the sky
that holds them
as it holds me,
& I'd say
joyfully,
namaste.

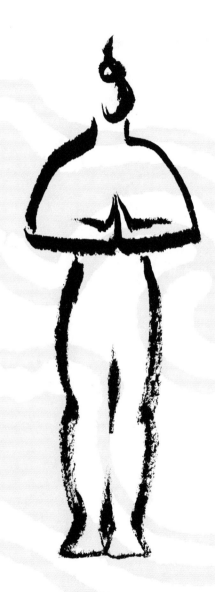

Surya Namascar

SUN SALUTATION

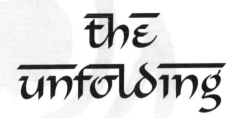

the
unfolding

Parighasana

BEAM USED FOR SHUTTING A GATE

A thousand fence posts
marching to the west
like teeth fixed
on the earth
mouths open into
mist-clouds
approaching the
ocean
raised in high tide
like an eyebrow
Chinese painting of the
Sung Dynasty
early morning
fog
on
Valley Ford Road.

When I turned thirty
I climbed fences
every day
no longer wanting
to build them.

Halasana

PLOUGH

The basket my great-great grandfather
carried on his back from Odessa
a linen tablecloth
silver samovar
brass candlesticks
for the Sabbath
hidden inside.
Its weave is still strong.
Its hinges still open and close.
It holds wood near the fireplace
and the wood keeps me warm.

I think I resemble it now,
my head tucked under
my legs
extended over it,
past and future folding into one.
He was once the son of Samuel,
grandson to a man, also Samuel
but my great-great-grandfather's name
was shortened to make it
easy to say in America.
All I ever knew of him
was this basket
and one word: peasant.

I don't know the name
of the person next to me
bending his body
in this free land
where the earth we plough
is the resistance to others.

Padahastasana

STANDING FOOT ON HANDS

It was somewhere on my heel,
that she knew.
Soft round swell of skin
puffed out like a sail,
my sister, homeopathic doctor,
old-soul, diviner of feet,
said I was with child.
But when I tried to find the child in me
I couldn't until a month
and many distractions later,
when another woman passed her hands
across my belly
and asked me quietly what had happened
to the soul of my son.

I thought back to that night in Tokyo
doubled over
(and here the doubled means both half and two)
in pain, unlike the usual monthly discomforts
and I knew then
that his soul had spilled out
and into the dark geography
within me
like a lighthouse beam
cutting across a starless night.
I never looked up and saw it.

Caught up in the rush
of another language
and the loss of my own,
caught up in the beauty of
falling cherry blossom leaves

and the pulse of subways and meetings
I didn't stop to feel the loss,
thought perhaps I'd imagined it all
at the hands of healers
until that afternoon in Marin City
bending over to slide the palms
of my hands
under the souls of my feet
facing Daissy,
herself an exile from a foreign land
who knew what might have been
when she touched my belly.

If the soul of my son
had indeed left my body weeks before,
it had not really entered
it until that day back in California
when I came home to
float in a bath of Dead Sea salts
the arms of my lover around me,
finally rising naked at the snap
of a branch in the backyard
where a trio of deer
had come to eat the bay laurel,
the small buck
at the picture window
staring straight out at
our still-dripping figures
having not yet
learned the fear of humans,
his ears twitching
at the sound of a distant car
on the road up above.

THE UNFOLDING

Surya Namascar

SUN SALUTATION

Everything she touches
turns to gold.
They say that now.
They didn't know her then.
She spent the first twelve years
of her life locked in a closet
and the next twelve
trying to break down the doors
that were no longer there.
She learned that nothing changes
but the changed.
She has all the character one gets
from suffering.
She is tired of suffering.
She is tired of telling her story.
She's survived.
Now she just wants to live.
She knows that Midas died
broken and weak.
She knows you can't live on gold.
All she wants to do is
touch the sun.

Purvottanasana

EAST STRETCH

My heart has been East
        when my body's been West.
My body's been East
        when my heart has been West.
My heart has been East
        when my body's been East
But my heart has not been West
        when my body's been West.

        Until now,
when somehow
        East and West
meet in the mirror,
        and the beloved earth
and I become one.

Utkatasana

CHAIR

You look just like her, the painter says,
lifting his brush to the canvas.
In the portrait,
the woman's eyes

are cold but real.
To look into them
is to swim into a wave
that sweeps you up in its power.
The one thing staring out

of the blue portrait
is the apple-bright red
of the woman's lips
parted slightly around unspoken words.

Sit down, he said, *and I'll paint you.*
She doesn't feel like
the woman at all.
In her own mind's eye
she is the artist, still unborn.

Years later,
no longer the artist's model,
she sits
on an imaginary chair
that cannot break
because it is composed
of her own power.
How long can she sit still
for herself?

And then,
a poem is born
in her body,
motion from stillness,
when entering
not striking
a pose.

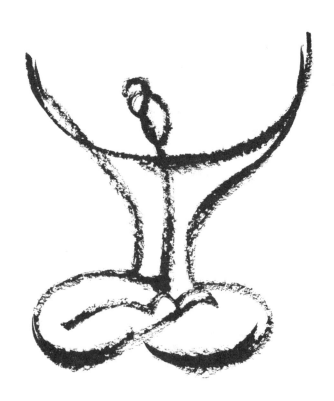

notes

p. 32 From *Yoga Sutra*, "Kaivalyapada," Verse 4.29: "There arises a state of mind full of clarity concerning all things at all times. It is like a rainfall of pure clarity."

p. 38 This poem is written to a lover who has died. Lazarus is the figure in the Bible (John 11:41–44) whom Jesus raises from the dead. St. Lazarus reportedly fled to Provence, where he later was presumed to have become the first bishop of Marseilles. He was imprisoned and beheaded in the second half of the first century. This poem was also inspired by Sylvia Plath's "Lady Lazarus."

p. 50 Siva (also Shiva) is the third god of the Hindu Trinity, the god of destruction. The Hindu trinity is composed of Brahma, the Creator; Vishnu, the Maintainer; and Siva, the destroyer of the universe.

Parvati is the goddess who was Siva's lover.

pp. 55, 68 Italicized four-line poems by Kijima Hajime, part of a form he created in which two or more poets may create chains of Linked Quatrains by following either of the two rules below:

1. Choose a word (or phrase) from the third line of another poet's quatrain. Use either its antonym or its synonym in the third line of your new quatrain.

2. Choose a word (or phrase) from the fourth line of another poet's quatrain. Use that same word (phrase) in the first line of your new quatrain.

The only other rule is that each poem must consist of four lines. Line length, meter, rhyme, et al., are wide open.

p. 65 Quan Yin is the Chinese goddess of mercy and healing, the bodhisattva of compassion. She is called Kannon in Japanese and Avalokitesvara in Sanskrit.

p. 68 This poem refers to the thousand-handed Kannon in religious depictions.

p. 69 Yasunari Kawabata, one of Japan's most distinguished postwar novelists, received the 1968 Nobel Prize for Literature and died in 1972 by his own hand. As a boy he had wanted to become a painter, and his novels and short stories are impressionistic and evocative. In 1923, he first began to write the highly condensed fictions he called "palm-of-the-hand stories."

p. 72 Ryoanji is a temple in Kyoto, site of a famous rock and sand Zen garden whose design dates back to around 1450. The garden's rocks are variously interpreted as being manifestations of infinity, islands in an ocean, part of the famous Inland Sea, or a mother tiger and her cubs. One can sit in front of the raked-sand masterpiece for hours and be transported.

p. 75 The Monkey story is as follows:

> Hanuman was the name of a powerful monkey chief of extraordinary strength and prowess. The son of Vayu, the god of Wind, and Anjana, he was the friend and dedicated servant of Rama, the seventh incarnation of Visnu. When Rama, his wife Sita, and his brother Laksmana were in exile as hermits in the Dandaka forest, Ravana, the demon king of Lanka (Ceylon), came to their hermitage in the guise of an ascetic and seizing Sita carried her off to Lanka while Rama and Laksmana were hunting game. The brothers searched far and wide for Sita, and enlisted the help of Sugriva, the king of the monkeys, and his general Hanuman. (B. K. S. Iyengar, *Light on Yoga*, p. 352)

<table>
<tr><td>p. 86</td><td>The Dead and The Dreamer are imagined archetypes. The poem was inspired by this quote from Carl Jung: "He who looks outside dreams, who looks inside wakes."</td></tr>
<tr><td>p. 99</td><td>*Namaste*: "I salute the light/god within."</td></tr>
</table>

The following works were consulted in the preparation of this book:

Feuerstein, Georg. *The Yoga Tradition: Its History, Literature, Philosophy, and Practice*. Prescott, Arizona: Hohm Press, 1998.

Iyengar, B. K. S. *Light on Yoga*. New York: Schocken Books, 1966, 1979.

Silva, Mira, and Shyam Mehta. *Yoga the Iyengar Way*. New York: Alfred A. Knopf, 1992.

Yoga, Discipline of Freedom: The Yoga Sutra Attributed to Patanjali. Translated by Barbara Stoler Miller. New York: Bantam Books, 1998.

"The Light of the Soul: The Yoga Sutra of Patanjali." Translated by the Tibetan Master Djwhal Kuhl. Commentary by Alice A. Bailey (www.spiritweb.org).

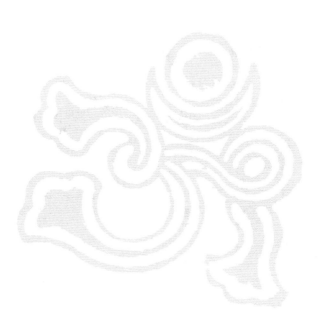

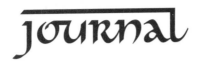

journal

Yoga awakens sensations in the body, opening the heart and mind to the infinite space without and within. It also invites emotions, memories, ideas, images, desires, and dreams to surface.

Keep this book beside you so that when you complete your practice, you can record what surfaces. How do you greet the "edge" of the blank page? Allow it to be a mirror, just like your yoga practice.

We often feel we cannot write "first drafts" in a new book or journal, as if the rawness of the words and emotions would somehow mar the book's beauty. Not so.

These pages offer the opportunity to allow yourself to write freely right now—without judging, striving to change, or editing your words. Unearthing your expression will cast light on it to help it grow.

Let your stories, like your body, begin to unfold.

116

117

118

DATE / LOCATION:

120

121

DATE / LOCATION:

122

DATE / LOCATION:

DATE / LOCATION: _____

_____

_____

_____

_____

_____

_____

_____

_____

_____

_____

_____

_____

_____

_____

_____

_____

_____

_____

_____

_____

125

_____

_____

_____

_____

DATE / LOCATION:

LEZA LOWITZ, a writer and student of Hatha yoga, trained at the White Lotus Foundation in Santa Barbara and now teaches yoga in northern California. She grew up in Berkeley and escaped to Tokyo, where she studied life, love, and Japanese in the secret capital. She is co-editor of two anthologies of contemporary Japanese women's poetry—*A Long Rainy Season* and *Other Side River* (Stone Bridge Press)—and author of a volume of poetry, *Old Ways to Fold New Paper* (Wandering Mind). Her honors include the PEN Syndicated Fiction Award and the Benjamin Franklin Award for Editorial Excellence, as well as grants from the National Endowment for the Arts, the National Endowment for the Humanities, and the California Arts Council. She is currently Co-Chair of the Marin Poetry Center and lives on the coast north of San Francisco with her Japanese husband and ninja dog. One day she hopes to be able to do *Gomukhasana* (Cow-Faced Pose) on both sides.

ANJA BORGSTROM is a yoga teacher, painter, printmaker, book-binder, and note-card designer based in Berkeley, California. In 1998 she started Ground Spirit Images, which represents her yoga-inspired art and allows her two careers—artist and yoga teacher—to complement each other. She exhibits her work annually at the Yoga, Mind, Spirit Conference in Estes Park, Colorado, and also on an ongoing basis throughout the San Francisco Bay Area. Her work is figurative, colorful, and textural, and often portrays energetic, ecstatic, or meditative yoga postures. These yogic figures represent awakening, contemplation, inquiry, nurturing of the feminine, and honoring of earth and spirit.